PLANTAR FASCIITIS

A Comprehensive Guide to Heel Pain

What is going on with my heel?

Mr Ewan Kannegieter
MSc FRCPodS FFPM RCPS (Glasg)

Edition number 1.0

Book ISBN 978-1-9193356-0-5

This publication is for general information and educational purposes only and is not a substitute for professional medical advice. Always consult a qualified healthcare professional regarding any medical condition.

Contents

Author's Foreword

Plantar heel pain is common, frustrating, and frequently misunderstood. Despite a strong evidence base supporting conservative, load-informed management, patients are often exposed to conflicting advice, premature escalation, and unnecessary investigations.

This guide provides a clear, balanced, evidence based explanation of plantar heel pain for patients, grounded in contemporary clinical guidelines and real world clinical practice. It emphasises diagnosis through history and examination, proportionate use of imaging, and the central role of education, load management, footwear, and progressive exercise.

Importantly, it avoids over-medicalisation and false promises. Instead, it offers patients a coherent framework for understanding their symptoms and engaging with recovery in a realistic and structured way. As such, this guide is intended to sit comfortably alongside appropriate clinical care.

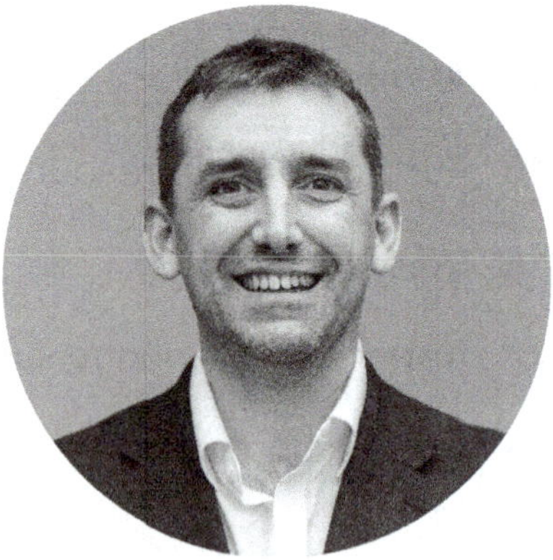

1. Introduction

What is going on with my heel?

Plantar fasciitis is one of the most common causes of heel pain. It accounts for the majority of non-traumatic heel pain seen in adults. It occurs when the thick band of tissue under your foot, the plantar fascia, becomes overloaded, irritated, or develops small tears near its attachment to the heel bone.

The classic story is sharp, stabbing, or aching heel pain with the first steps out of bed or after sitting for a while. It often eases as you move, but can return with activity or by the end of the day. Around one third of people experience symptoms in both feet.

> It's very common. Roughly one in ten people will experience it at some point in their lives, most often between ages 40 and 60, but it can affect younger and older people too.

A candid note from clinic

If you are reading this with that familiar first step pain, you are not imagining it. The pain can be surprisingly sharp and demoralising, particularly because it often improves as you walk, only to return later. That up-and-down pattern can be extremely frustrating.

A helpful way to think about plantar heel pain is that your tissue capacity has been exceeded. Something has changed, sometimes obviously, sometimes subtly: your step count crept up, you returned to running, you stood more at work, you changed shoes, you gained a bit of weight, your calf muscles tightened, you had an injury and altered your walking. The fascia does not fail because it is delicate. It fails because the load exceeded what it could tolerate at that time.

Good news: when you understand the drivers, the plan is usually straightforward. It is not magic. It is load management, support, plus progressive strengthening, done consistently.

This guide reflects the same conversations I have every week in clinic with people struggling with heel pain. While many readers will recover using the information here alone, some will benefit from individual assessment and guidance.

What this guide will do:

- Help you recognise the usual pattern of plantar heel pain
- Give you a practical plan that is realistic, not perfect
- Explain what tends to work, and why
- Show you when it is time to get help and what the next steps look like

What this guide will not do:

- Promise a cure in a week
- Tell you that one gadget will fix it
- Pretend every heel pain is plantar fasciitis

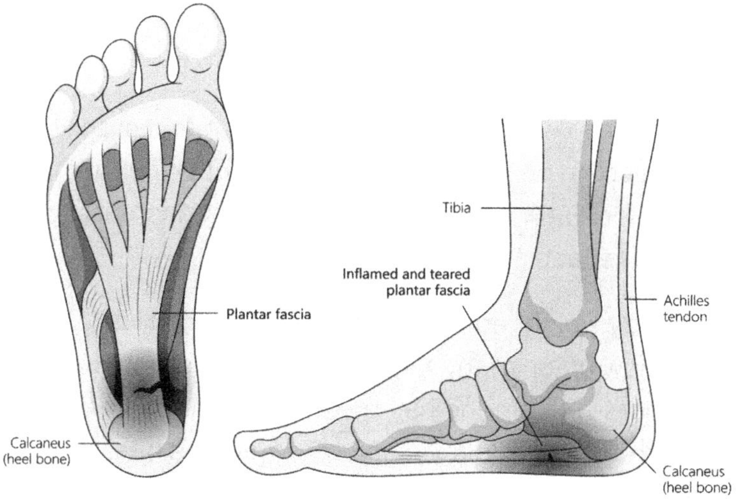

2. Causes and risk factors

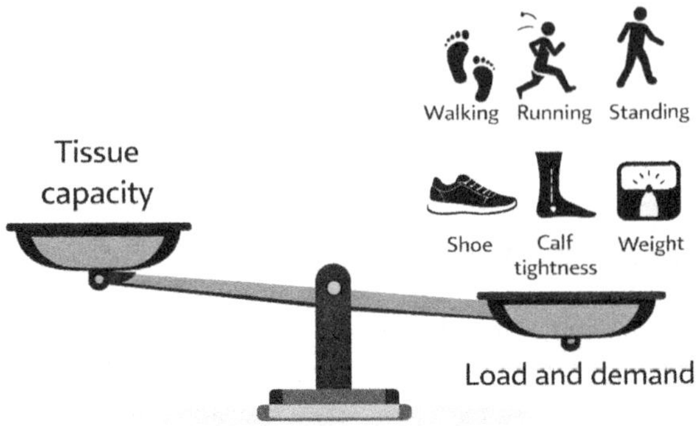

Plantar fasciitis is usually the result of repeated stress and strain. Standing all day on hard floors, sudden increases in exercise, or taking on more than your body is ready for can all tip the balance.

Certain job roles are more prone to heel pain, including hairdressers, chefs, nurses, police officers, and anyone on their feet for long shifts.

Very flat feet, very high arches, or reduced foot stability can increase strain on the plantar fascia. Tight calf or hamstring muscles, or a stiff Achilles tendon, can also increase load through the fascia.

Extra body weight adds load to each step, and while heel spurs show up on many X-rays, they are often innocent bystanders with around half the population having a heel spur without issue. In my opinion, removing a heel spur rarely solves plantar fasciitis.

> Most cases come down to a common issue: the fascia is being stressed faster than it can heal, creating a cycle of irritation and pain.

What that actually means in real life

Repeated stress and strain is a bland phrase, so let's put it into day-to-day examples.

Common triggers I hear in clinic

- New job, longer shifts, more standing on hard floors
- A sudden return to exercise, especially running, hills, or high intensity classes
- A change in footwear, often to something flatter, softer, or more worn out than you realise
- A holiday with far more walking than usual
- A period of reduced activity followed by a rapid ramp up.

Common background factors

- Calf and hamstring tightness that has gradually increased over time
- Foot motion that is greater or less than average can alter how load travels through the arch.

- A slightly shorter stride or altered gait due to hip, knee, or back pain
- Weight change, even modest, because every extra kilogram multiplies through thousands of steps.

Body weight and plantar heel pain

Body weight deserves a fuller explanation, as it is one of the most consistent risk factors for plantar heel pain and is often oversimplified.

A higher body mass index (BMI) is a well-established independent risk factor for plantar fasciitis. Observational studies and systematic reviews show a stepwise increase in risk as BMI rises, with higher BMI categories associated with substantially greater odds of plantar heel pain. This association is particularly strong in non-athletic populations, where training load is less likely to be the primary driver.

The explanation is largely mechanical. Each step places load through the plantar fascia; as body weight increases, that load increases proportionally across thousands of steps per day. Over time, this can exceed the tissue's capacity to adapt, leading to damage and gradual collagen degeneration at the fascia's attachment to the heel.

Imaging and biomechanical studies support this pattern. In plantar heel pain, the plantar fascia often becomes thicker but less resilient. Rather than being stronger, the tissue absorbs load less efficiently and is more prone to irritation. These changes are characteristic of plantar fasciopathy rather than healthy adaptation. Put simply, the tissue is being asked to do more work, more often, with less opportunity to recover between loads.

It is important to be clear about what this does and does not mean. Plantar fasciitis is not exclusive to people with higher body weight, and many individuals of healthy or normal weight develop plantar heel pain, particularly in association with changes in activity, footwear, or calf flexibility. Body weight is not a judgement, and it is rarely the only factor involved. Many people with higher BMI never develop heel pain, and many people with plantar fasciitis are not overweight. What matters is the interaction between load, recovery, footwear, calf flexibility, activity levels, and foot mechanics. Body weight is one contributor within that wider system.

When it comes to treatment, the picture is more nuanced. Clinical guidelines recognise the strong association between higher BMI and chronic plantar heel pain, but evidence that modest weight loss alone leads to rapid pain relief is limited. Exercise remains central to management, but its benefit comes primarily from targeted stretching and strengthening rather than weight reduction itself.

More substantial and sustained weight loss appears to have a clearer effect. Studies following bariatric surgery show marked reductions in foot pain, improved mobility, and reduced healthcare use for plantar fasciitis, with many patients reporting symptom resolution. This supports the idea that reducing mechanical load at scale can meaningfully change the load environment experienced by the plantar fascia.

For most people, the practical takeaway is this: weight management can be a helpful supporting strategy, but it is rarely a standalone solution. The most effective approach combines load management, supportive footwear, progressive strengthening, and realistic activity pacing. Where weight reduction is appropriate and achievable, it may improve outcomes over time and reduce the risk of recurrence, but it should sit within a broader, compassionate management plan rather than being presented as the sole answer.

The heel spur myth

Many people are told they have a heel spur and assume it is the cause. In reality, spurs are common in people with no symptoms, and many people with classic plantar heel pain have no spur. Spurs often represent long-term traction change at the heel rather than the source of pain. The focus should typically stay on the fascia and the load environment.

A simple rule that helps

If your heel pain began after a clear change in routine, your plan should include reversing some of that change temporarily, then rebuilding gradually. If your heel pain began with no obvious trigger, it is usually still load related, but the trigger is often hidden in the background: a gradual change in calf muscle flexibility, worn footwear, more standing, less sleep, more stress, or a quiet increase in daily steps.

3. Signs and symptoms

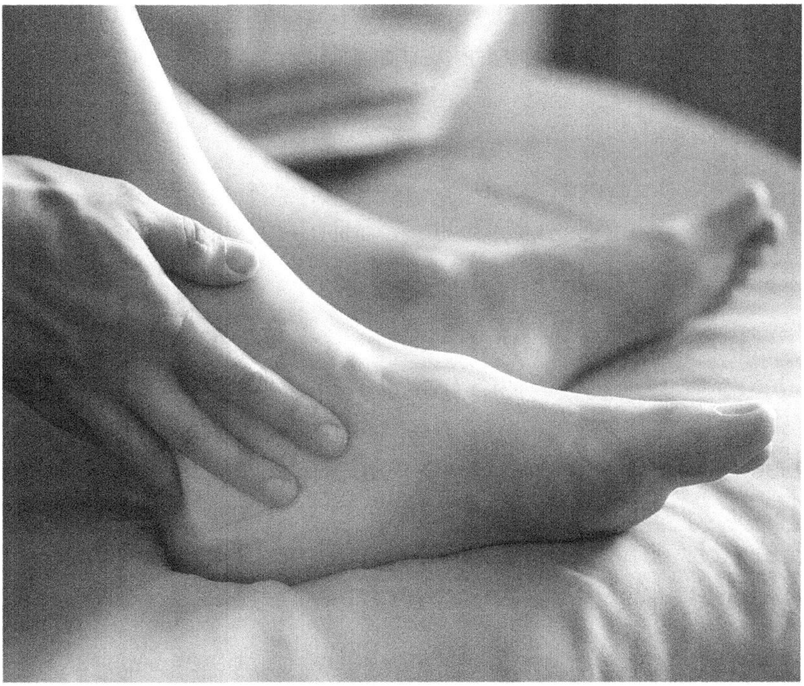

Plantar fasciitis often develops gradually, though sometimes it can appear quite suddenly after a change in activity, footwear, or routine.

- Pain is usually under the heel, sometimes spreading into the arch
- It is typically worse with first steps in the morning or after rest

- Pressing the bottom of the heel often reproduces the pain
- The pain usually eases with movement, but can return with prolonged standing, walking, or sport.

It usually does not cause swelling, redness, tingling or numbness. If those are present, another problem may be at play and should be checked.

Because the symptoms are distinctive, podiatrists typically diagnose plantar fasciitis based on history and examination alone. Imaging is not always required, but ultrasound can be useful, particularly for assessing plantar fascia thickness and comparing it with normal values. X-ray can be used to rule out stress fractures, or MRI for bone marrow oedema if the case is atypical or not improving.

Imaging is often more useful for ruling out other causes of heel pain than for confirming plantar fasciitis itself. Imaging findings should always be interpreted alongside symptoms, not in isolation.

A little more nuance, when to pause and reconsider the diagnosis

Most cases are straightforward, but a minority are not. Consider getting assessed sooner if any of these fit:

- Pain that is constant at rest, occurs at night, or wakes you from sleep
- Pins and needles, burning, numbness, or pain that shoots into the arch or toes
- Significant swelling, heat, redness, or fever
- Pain mainly at the back of the heel, which is more often Achilles-related
- A history of inflammatory arthritis, gout, or recent infection
- Diabetes with reduced sensation or known circulation problems

Some alternatives include heel fat pad pain, a calcaneal stress fracture, or nerve irritation such as Baxter's nerve entrapment. The point is not to worry you, but to avoid months of self-care for the wrong problem.

4. Understanding the plantar fascia: why load matters

The plantar fascia is a thick band of connective tissue that runs from the heel bone to the toes. It helps support the arch and helps the foot become a stable lever when you push off.

A key concept is the windlass mechanism. When the toes bend upwards, the fascia tightens, which helps lift and stiffen the arch. This is normal. The issue is not movement itself, but repetition without adequate recovery. The problem occurs when the fascia is repeatedly asked to absorb more load than it can tolerate.

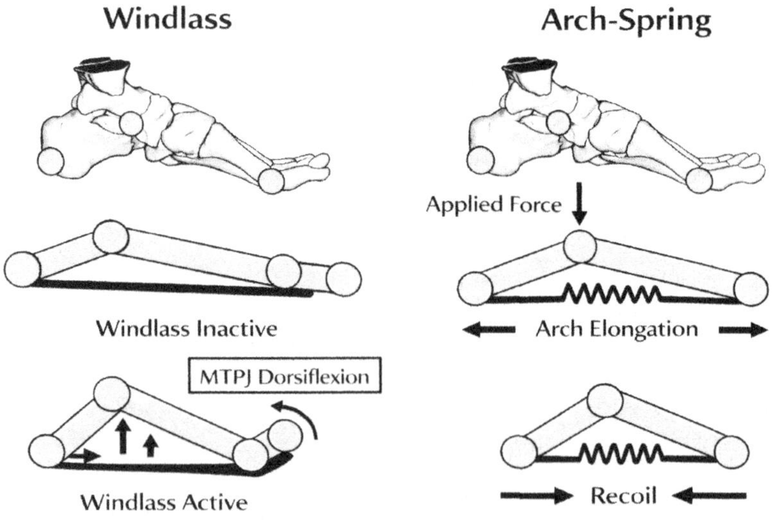

Three common load amplifiers:

- Limited ankle dorsiflexion due to tight calf muscles or Achilles stiffness
- Prolonged standing, especially on hard surfaces
- Foot posture and gait patterns such as very flat feet (pes planus), or very high arches (pes cavus)

If you only remember one biomechanics point, remember this: you do not need perfect feet to recover. You need a plan that reduces overload and rebuilds capacity.

---

5. Conservative treatment, first-line care

Conservative treatment involves a combination of low risk measures that reduce strain on the plantar fascia and allow recovery. These include rest and pacing, ice, short term pain relief if appropriate, supportive footwear, insoles or heel cups, cushioned mats, and progressive stretching and load management.

The good news is that most people get better without surgery. But it takes patience: months rather than weeks.

Here are the mainstays of treatment:

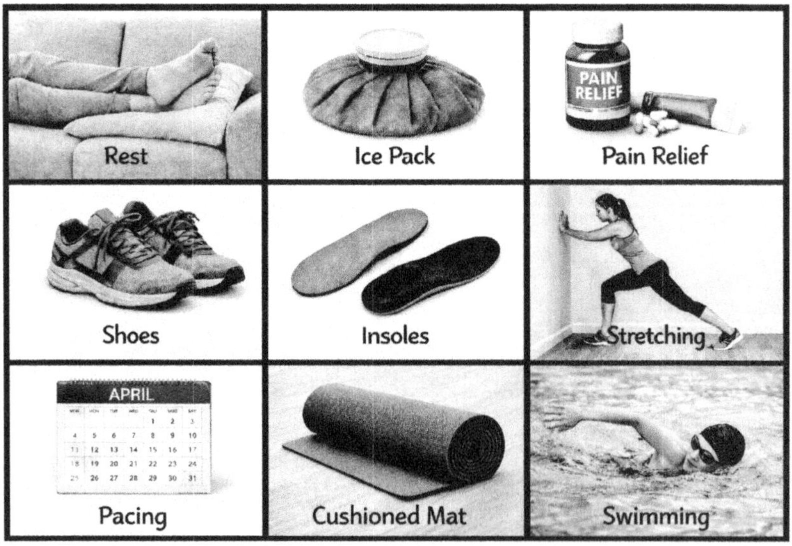

Rest and activity modification

Take pressure off the heel. If able, swap running for cycling or swimming. Break up long standing periods if you can. Small changes reduce irritation and give the fascia a chance to calm down.

Practical examples that actually help:

- Split a long walk into two shorter walks
- Use a cushioned mat at a standing desk or in the kitchen
- Avoid barefoot walking on hard floors, especially first thing in the morning. Instead keep supportive, thick-soled shoes or sneakers by the bed
- Reduce hills and speed work if you run
- Reduce standing still, gentle walking is often better than prolonged static standing

Ice and pain relief

Ice packs, or rolling your heel over a frozen water bottle for around 10 minutes, can help ease pain after activity. Simple anti-inflammatory medication, such as ibuprofen, may also help if it is safe for you and used according to advice or packaging. This can be taken orally or applied as a topical gel, but it should be viewed as short-term symptom relief rather than a long-term solution.

Pain relief is not cheating. It is a tool. The aim is to help you stay functional while you rebuild your tolerance.

Stretching

Regular, focused stretching of the plantar fascia, calf muscles, and hamstrings is one of the most effective remedies for heel pain. With so many different exercises available, it can feel overwhelming. My advice is simple: choose one exercise, do it well, and do it often.

For example, to stretch calf and hamstring muscles on the painful side:

- Sit with the affected leg stretched out straight, knee locked
- Bend the other knee so that foot rests flat on the surface; sofa, bed, or floor
- Keeping the knee straight on the stretched side, bend your ankle so your toes point upwards, towards the ceiling, or ideally slightly back towards you
- You may feel tightness behind the leg and an urge to bend the knee; try to resist this
- To deepen the stretch, lean forwards and reach both hands towards the toes of the affected foot, keeping the knee straight and the toes gently drawn back towards you
- Hold for 10 seconds, then relax. Aim for several short sessions across the day, totalling around 5 to 7 minutes of stretching per day
- Consistency matters. Daily stretching over several weeks produces the best long-term results

6. Exercise therapy in detail, stretching and strengthening

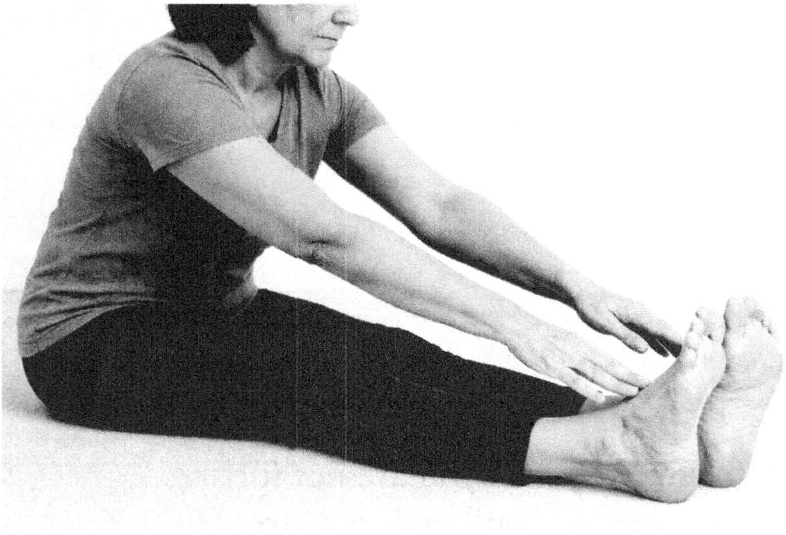

Stretching reduces tension. Strengthening rebuilds capacity. Both matter, but they do different jobs.

What are we actually trying to strengthen?

In plantar heel pain, the goal is not to "strengthen the plantar fascia directly" in the way you might strengthen a muscle. The plantar fascia is a tough connective tissue. It adapts slowly and responds best when the forces passing through it are better controlled.

That control comes from three main areas:

- The calf and Achilles tendon, which regulate how much force reaches the heel with each step
- The small intrinsic muscles of the foot, which help support the arch during standing and walking
- The overall loading pattern, including how quickly and how often force is applied

When these systems are weak or poorly conditioned, the plantar fascia is asked to do more work than it can tolerate. Strengthening shifts load away from the fascia and improves how force is absorbed and released.

In simple terms: you are not forcing the fascia to "bulk up", you are building a stronger, more efficient support system around it.

Why stretching alone is often not enough

Stretching is excellent for reducing morning pain and easing tension, particularly if the hamstrings, calf or Achilles are tight. For many people, this brings early improvement.

However, stretching does not restore load tolerance.

This is why some people plateau: the pain settles a little, but the tissue still cannot cope with normal daily demands. Without strengthening, the same overload cycle continues.

When to start strengthening

Strengthening is not about pushing through pain. It is about reintroducing load in a controlled way.

You can usually begin gentle strengthening when:

- Morning pain is no longer a sharp 9 out of 10
- Pain does not spike dramatically the day after normal daily activities
- Small increases in activity do not trigger a major flare

Some discomfort during exercises is acceptable. Sharp pain, or pain that steadily worsens week by week, is not.

What strengthening should focus on

1. Calf strength (most important)

Calf raises are the foundation.

- Start with double-leg calf raises, holding a support
- Progress slowly before attempting single-leg work
- Move through a comfortable range, controlled up and down

This is often the single most important strengthening exercise for plantar heel pain.

2. Foot intrinsic muscle strength

The small muscles within the foot help stabilise the arch during stance and push-off. When they are weak, the plantar fascia takes on more strain.

Simple exercises include:

- Short foot exercises (raising the arch without curling the toes)
- Gentle toe control exercises

These are subtle exercises. Quality matters more than effort.

3. Load progression, not exhaustion

The aim is not fatigue for its own sake. The aim is gradual exposure to load, allowing tissues time to adapt.

Think in terms of:

- Consistency over weeks
- Small increases, not sudden jumps
- Monitoring how the foot feels the next morning

If symptoms are improving overall, you are on the right track.

How stretching and strengthening work together

- Stretching reduces resting tension and morning pain
- Strengthening improves how load is managed during the day
- Together, they increase the margin between what the tissue can tolerate and what it is being asked to do

This is how recovery becomes durable, not just temporary.

A realistic expectation

Improvement is rarely linear. There will be good days and frustrating ones. What matters is the overall trend.

If you feel:

- Fewer bad mornings
- Shorter flares
- More confidence in your foot

Then the programme is working.

If progress stalls despite consistent, well-applied exercise, that is the point at which individual review can help refine the plan.

7. Footwear, insoles, splints and taping

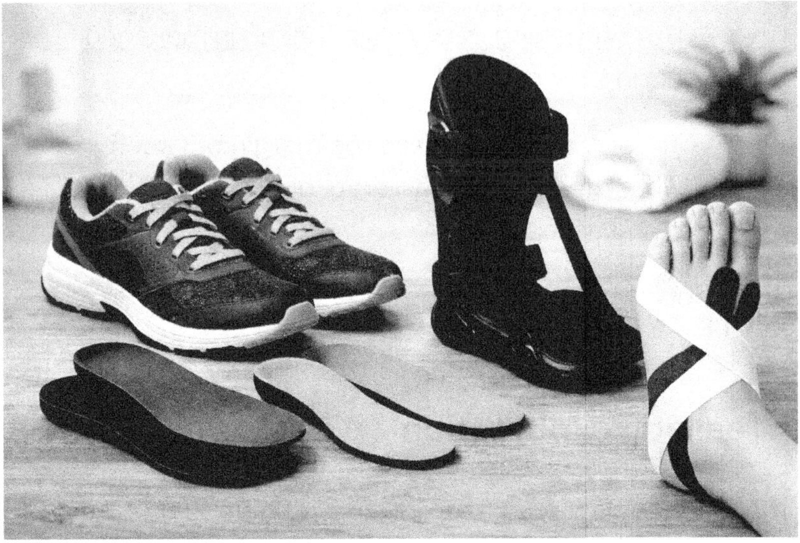

Shoes matter. Avoid flimsy footwear or going barefoot on hard floors. Supportive trainers or shoes with thick cushioning protect the heel.

Footwear and orthotics

Footwear that works well for heel pain is usually stable rather than soft or floppy. Shoes with a firm heel counter, good midsole support, and cushioning under the heel help reduce repeated impact and limit excessive strain through the plantar fascia. Very flexible shoes, worn-out trainers, flip-flops, and thin-soled footwear often allow symptoms to persist or worsen.

Over-the-counter insoles, heel cups, or arch supports, often 15 to 40 pounds or 20 to 50 dollars, can significantly reduce heel pain. They are relatively inexpensive and can be swapped between shoes.

Tip: Keep supportive shoes by the bed. Stretch first, then slip them on before those painful first steps.

Night splints or socks

These keep the foot gently stretched overnight. They are particularly helpful if mornings are your worst time. Boot styles exist, but soft sock versions, like a Strassburg sock, are less bulky. Wearing them for 1 to 3 months can make a big difference.

Taping

Taping can be a useful short term tool, especially on high step days or long shifts. If taping helps, ask a podiatrist or physiotherapist to teach you a method you can repeat reliably.

Custom orthotics

If simple insoles help but do not go far enough, or if your biomechanics are clearly contributing, custom orthoses can be useful. They should feel like a steering correction, not a rigid cast. Custom devices should always sit alongside exercise and load management, not replace them

8. A six-week plan and when to get help

Recovery from plantar fasciitis takes time, consistency, and a bit of patience.

For most people, the pain improves with simple steps done regularly at home, but progress can feel slow at first. This six-week guide sets out a clear, realistic plan showing what to focus on at each stage, how to build up activity safely, and when to seek professional help if your heel pain is not settling as expected.

Weeks 1 to 2:

Rest, ice, stretch, supportive shoes, insoles. Avoid high impact activity.

Weeks 3 to 4:

If mornings are still rough, add a night splint. Keep stretching. Start strengthening exercises.

Weeks 5 to 6:

If improving, gradually reintroduce walking or low impact activity. If not improving, this is a sensible point to check in with a podiatrist.

Seek help sooner if pain is worsening, constant even at rest, or comes with redness, swelling, or nerve symptoms.

Making this plan work in the real world

This is where people either progress or drift. Here is how I encourage you to run the plan.

Pick two lead measures

- Morning first step pain out of 10
- Total steps per day, even roughly

Then adjust one thing at a time.

If you change shoes, add insoles, start stretching, start strengthening, start night splints, and start shockwave all at once, you will never know what helped and what irritated you.

What improvement looks like

Improvement is not always pain free. It is fewer bad mornings, less sharpness, shorter flares, and a gradual return of confidence.

Red flags that need reassessment

- No improvement at all after six weeks of consistent basics
- Any suggestion of nerve symptoms
- Pain that has moved, changed character, or become more constant

Plateaus are common and do not mean failure.

When individual advice may help

If your pain is not improving despite consistent self-care, or if you are unsure whether your symptoms truly fit plantar heel pain, an in-person assessment can be valuable.

9. Imaging, what it can and cannot tell you

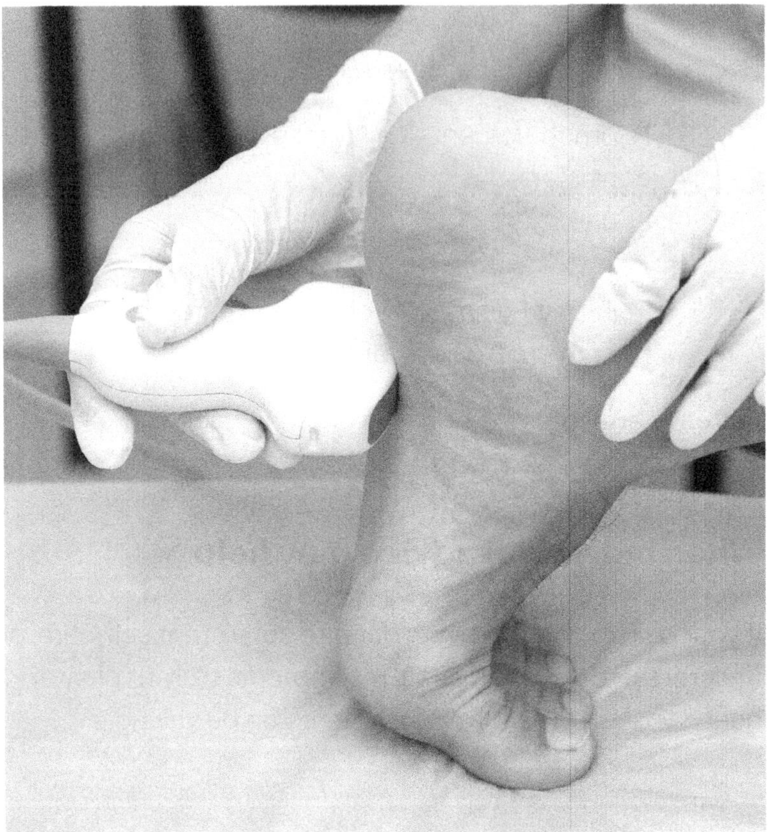

Imaging is not always required. A good clinical history and examination often gets you most of the way there.

When imaging can help:

- Symptoms are not typical
- There is concern about stress fracture, nerve entrapment, or another diagnosis
- Symptoms persist despite good quality conservative care
- You need reassurance, or clarity for return to activity decisions

What each modality can do:

- **X-ray**, useful to rule out bony pathology, spurs may be present but are not the cause
- **Ultrasound**, shows fascia thickness and tissue change, can guide injections when required
- **MRI**, used for atypical or non-improving cases, can assess bone marrow oedema and soft tissue detail

10. Advanced treatments

If six weeks or more of consistent self-care has not resolved symptoms, podiatrists can offer further options:

- Custom orthotics
- Shockwave therapy
- Corticosteroid injections
- Boot immobilisation
- Surgery, rare

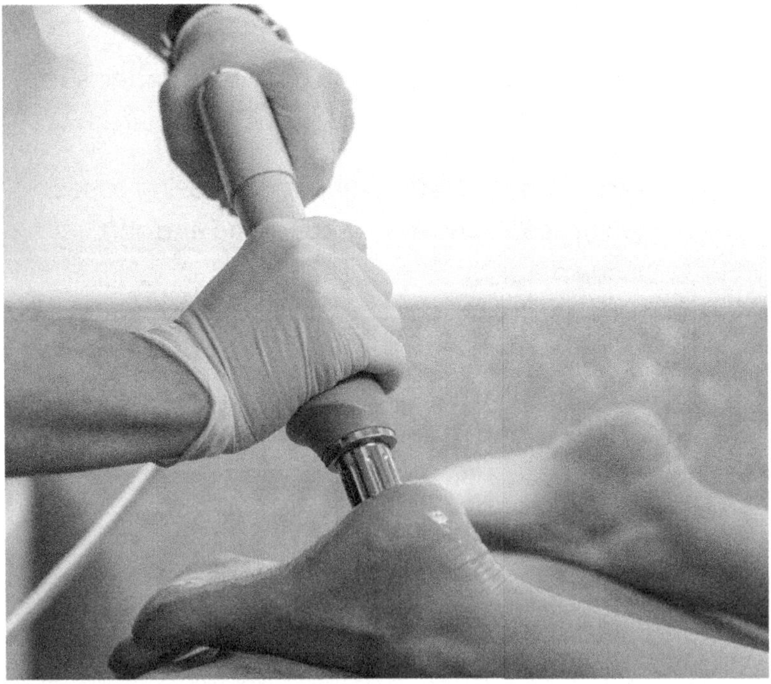

How to think about advanced treatments

The goal is not to collect treatments, but to use the right tool at the right time within an overall load and recovery plan.

Steroid injections can be useful when pain is blocking rehabilitation, but they should not be the only plan. If you get pain relief and then go straight back to your previous load, relapse is common.

Shockwave is often a sensible next step in a stubborn case, particularly when there is a clear diagnosis, persistent symptoms, and a good foundation of self-care. It can be a bridge that reduces pain enough for proper progressive loading. Response is often gradual over weeks rather than immediate.

Boot immobilisation can calm symptoms, but it can also weaken the calf if overused. If you use a boot, plan the exit and the rebuild at the same time.

Custom orthoses are most helpful when your mechanics are clearly contributing and when simple insoles have not been enough. They should feel like a steering wheel correction, not a rigid brace.

Layering depth, what clinicians tend to do, and why that matters

A useful observation from the UK is that plantar heel pain is managed across different professional groups, including podiatrists, physiotherapists, orthotists, GPs, and others.

A UK survey of registered healthcare professionals reported that education, exercise based approaches, and prefabricated orthoses are commonly used, with variation in how and when more advanced options are chosen.

From a patient point of view, that means two things:

1. If you have seen one clinician and not improved, it does not automatically mean you are stuck. It may mean the plan has not yet matched your drivers.
2. You want a plan that is coherent. Support the heel, calm symptoms, then build strength and tolerance. If you jump between ten different treatments without a strategy, you can lose months.

11. Surgery, rare but real, what it actually involves

Surgery is considered only if everything else fails after six to twelve months of comprehensive non-surgical care.

Plantar fascia release

One procedure option is a plantar fasciotomy; a partial release of the plantar fascia. It can be done endoscopically, through a small scope, or via a small open incision.

Surgical outcomes with this approach are not guaranteed. Estimates suggest surgery is required in a small minority (<5–10%) of patients, and some of them may still have pain afterward or develop complications, including tightness of the remaining portions of the plantar fascia following this procedure, nerve injury and potential changes in foot architecture leading to flat foot.

A clinician's explanation:

The decision for surgery is about time, function, and the quality of the conservative programme already tried. It is not about being brave or desperate.

If surgery is on the table, it is worth ensuring that calf tightness has been assessed properly, that the diagnosis is correct, and that the rehabilitation plan is realistic. In many cases, the issue is not that conservative care failed, but that it was incomplete or inconsistent.

Gastrocnemius recession

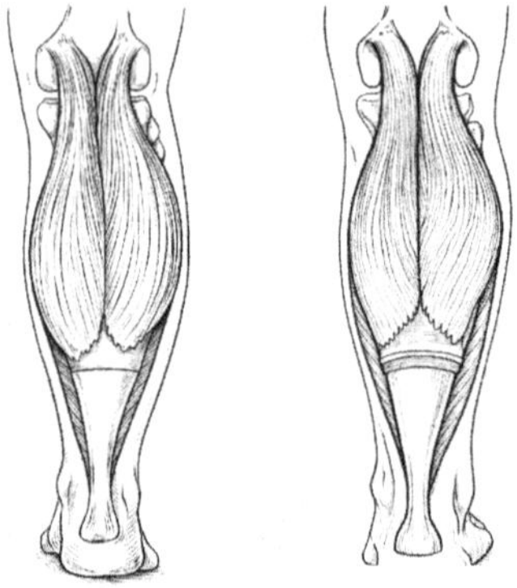

For some, the real culprit is not just the fascia but tight calf muscles, specifically the gastrocnemius. When these muscles are too tight, the ankle cannot bend upwards properly, piling stress on the fascia.

If stretching and footwear do not solve this, podiatric surgeons including myself sometimes recommend a gastrocnemius recession.

What happens:

- A small incision is made at the back of the lower leg
- The fascia around the gastrocnemius muscle is released, lengthening the muscle tendon unit
- This frees up ankle movement and reduces strain on the fascia

Why it is done:

- Persistent plantar fasciitis with proven calf tightness
- Sometimes used for Achilles problems, forefoot overload, or as part of flatfoot correction

Benefits:

- Looser calf, easier ankle movement
- Reduced heel pain

- No direct action or scarring of the Achilles
- Often a day case procedure

Risks:

- Temporary calf weakness
- Scar or indentation at the back of the leg
- Sural nerve irritation; numbness on outer side of the foot
- Recurrence of calf tightness over time

Recovery:

- Often involves a boot and crutches for around 2 weeks, with weight bearing progressed gradually from week 2 to 6 with physiotherapy rehab
- Walking more normally at 6 to 8 weeks

Bottom line: This is a specialist option, reserved for the few who do not improve with comprehensive nonsurgical care.

---

12. Prognosis and prevention

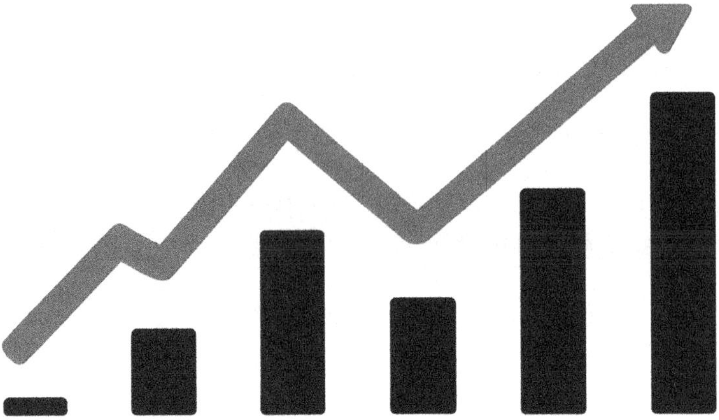

The outlook is generally positive with plantar fasciitis. Around 80% improve significantly within 6 to 9 months, and about 90% are pain free within a year.

To prevent recurrence:

- Stick with supportive shoes and replace worn out trainers
- Do not ramp up running mileage too fast
- Keep up stretches for tight hamstrings and calf muscles
- Maintain a healthy body weight

- Do not ignore early twinges, catching it early saves months of trouble
- Always consider a podiatrist for foot pain advice

Why recurrence happens, and how to reduce it

Recurrence usually happens for the same reason it started: demand increases faster than capacity is rebuilt.

Setbacks do not mean you are back to the beginning; they usually respond faster with early adjustment.

> If you take one prevention concept away, it is this: keep a small amount of the boring basics in your routine even when you feel better. Two brief calf strengthening sessions a week, a few minutes of hamstring and calf stretching, and sensible footwear for high step days can keep your heel quiet.

If you are a runner, treat your calf muscles as part of your running engine. Strong calves reduce strain through the heel by sharing load properly. Also watch the obvious traps: sudden increases in hills, speed work, or long runs.

13. A note on clinical support

This book is designed to empower you with understanding and practical steps. It does not replace individual medical care, and some cases require tailored assessment.

Most people with plantar heel pain improve with consistent, well-applied conservative measures.

However, not all heel pain follows a straightforward course, and not all symptoms fit neatly into a single diagnosis. When pain persists despite good self-care, changes character, or begins to limit daily life more significantly, individual assessment can be valuable.

Clinical review allows the diagnosis to be confirmed, alternative causes of heel pain to be considered, and treatment to be adjusted to the specific factors driving symptoms. This may include review of activity levels, footwear, muscle tightness, foot mechanics, and, where appropriate, proportionate use of imaging or additional therapies.

Seeking clinical input is not a sign of failure or of having done anything wrong. It is simply part of matching the right level of care to the problem in front of you. Some people benefit from reassurance and refinement of a plan already in place; others benefit from targeted intervention when recovery has stalled. The aim, at every stage, is clarity: understanding what is happening, what matters most, and what the next sensible step should be.

14. About the Author

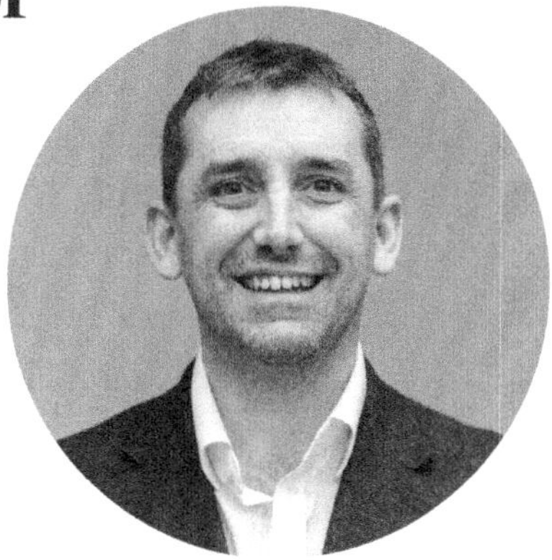

Mr Ewan Kannegieter MSc, FRCPodS, FFPM RCPS (Glasg) is a UK-trained Consultant Podiatric Surgeon and former Dean (2024–2026) of the Faculty of Podiatric Surgery at the Royal College of Podiatry. He leads Kann Foot Surgery Ltd and co-leads the Motion Clinic Group Ltd.

Ewan has played an active role in the training, governance, and development of podiatric surgery in the UK. He lectures nationally and internationally and serves as Adjunct Assistant Professor at the Frank H. Netter MD School of Medicine, Quinnipiac University (Connecticut, USA).

As a clinician, his focus is on helping people overcome foot and ankle pain through practical, evidence-based care, whether surgical, conservative, or focused on simple steps that support confident recovery.

Alongside his academic and leadership roles, Ewan continues to practise clinically, supporting patients with complex or persistent foot and ankle pain through clear diagnosis, proportionate investigation, and evidence-based care.

15. Further Resources

- **NHS England**
  – Plantar fasciitis: symptoms, causes, treatment and when to seek help
  https://www.nhs.uk/conditions/plantar-fasciitis/

- **Royal College of Podiatry**
  – Heel pain on the sole of the foot (plantar heel pain)
  https://www.rcpod.org.uk/heel-pain

- **American Podiatric Medical Association (APMA)**
  – Heel pain (plantar fasciitis)
  https://www.apma.org/heelpain

- **StatPearls (NCBI Bookshelf)**
  – Plantar fasciitis clinical overview
  https://www.ncbi.nlm.nih.gov/books/NBK431073/

- **JOSPT Clinical Practice Guideline (2023)**
  – Heel pain, plantar fasciitis
  https://www.jospt.org/doi/10.2519/jospt.2023.0303

- **Journal of Foot and Ankle Research (2025)**
  – UK survey of plantar heel pain management
  https://doi.org/10.1002/jfa2.70087

16. References

1. American Podiatric Medical Association (APMA). Heel pain (plantar fasciitis): patient information. https://www.apma.org/heelpain

2. Babatunde OO, Legha A, Littlewood C, et al. Comparative effectiveness of treatments for plantar heel pain: a systematic review with network meta-analysis. *British Journal of Sports Medicine.* 2019;53(3):182–194. https://doi.org/10.1136/bjsports-2017-098998

3. Boules M, Batayyah E, Froylich D, et al. Effect of surgical weight loss on plantar fasciitis and health care use. *Journal of the American Podiatric Medical Association.* 2018;108(6):442–448. https://doi.org/10.7547/15-169

4. Cooper MT. Common painful foot and ankle conditions: a review. *JAMA.* 2023;330(23):2285–2294. https://doi.org/10.1001/jama.2023.23906

5. Cotchett M, Rathleff MS, Dilnot M, et al. Lived experience of people with plantar heel pain: a qualitative study. *Journal of Foot and Ankle Research.* 2020;13:12. https://doi.org/10.1186/s13047-020-0378-9

6. Drake C, Chapman L, Burnett C, et al.
Plantar heel pain management: a survey of UK registered healthcare professionals.
Journal of Foot and Ankle Research.
2025;18:e70087.
https://doi.org/10.1002/jfa2.70087

7. Drake C, Whittaker GA, Kaminski MR, et al.
Medical imaging for plantar heel pain: a systematic review and meta-analysis.
Journal of Foot and Ankle Research. 2022;15:29.
https://doi.org/10.1186/s13047-022-00543-9

8. Hansen L, Krogh TP, Ellingsen T, Bolvig L, Fredberg U.
Long term prognosis of plantar fasciitis: a 5 to 15 year follow up study.
Orthopaedic Journal of Sports Medicine.
2018;6(3).
https://doi.org/10.1177/2325967118757983

9. Jha DK, Wongkaewpotong J, Chuckpaiwong B.
Effect of age and body mass index on sonographic findings of the plantar fascia.
Journal of Foot and Ankle Surgery.
2023;62(1):125–128.
https://doi.org/10.1053/j.jfas.2022.05.010

10. Journal of Orthopaedic and Sports Physical Therapy (JOSPT).
Heel pain plantar fasciitis: revision 2023. Clinical Practice Guideline.
https://www.jospt.org/doi/10.2519/jospt.2023.0303

11. Landorf KB, Kaminski MR, Munteanu SE, Zammit GV, Menz HB.
Health related quality of life in people with plantar heel pain.
Scientific Reports. 2022;12:16237.
https://doi.org/10.1038/s41598-022-20410-4

12. Menz HB, Jordan KP, Roddy E, Croft PR.
Characteristics of primary care consultations for musculoskeletal foot and ankle problems.
Rheumatology. 2010;49(7):1391–1398.
https://doi.org/10.1093/rheumatology/keq092

13. Morrissey D, Cotchett M, Said J'Bari A, et al.
Management of plantar heel pain: a best practice guide informed by a systematic review, expert clinical reasoning and patient values.
British Journal of Sports Medicine.
2021;55(19):1106–1118.
https://doi.org/10.1136/bjsports-2019-101970

14. NHS England.
Plantar fasciitis: symptoms, causes and treatment.
https://www.nhs.uk/conditions/plantar-fasciitis/

15. Riddle DL, Pulisic M, Pidcoe P, Johnson RE.
Risk factors for plantar fasciitis: a matched case control study.
Journal of Bone and Joint Surgery (American Volume). 2003;85(5):872–877.
https://doi.org/10.2106/00004623-200305000-00015

16. Royal College of Podiatry.
Heel pain on the sole of the foot (plantar heel pain): patient information.
https://www.rcpod.org.uk/heel-pain

17. StatPearls Publishing.
Plantar fasciitis. *NCBI Bookshelf.*
https://www.ncbi.nlm.nih.gov/books/NBK431073/

18. Taş S, Bek N, Onur MR, Korkusuz F.
Effects of body mass index on mechanical properties of the plantar fascia and heel pad in asymptomatic participants.
Foot and Ankle International. 2017;38(7):779–784.
https://doi.org/10.1177/1071100717702463

19. van Leeuwen KDB, Rogers J, Winzenberg T, van Middelkoop M.
Higher body mass index is associated with plantar fasciopathy: a systematic review and meta analysis.
British Journal of Sports Medicine.
2016;50(16):972–981.
https://doi.org/10.1136/bjsports-2015-095972

17. Appendix

Evidence Summary for Clinicians

Scope

This summary synthesises current evidence on plantar heel pain (PHP), commonly labelled plantar fasciitis, drawing on clinical guidelines, systematic reviews, epidemiological data, and patient-reported experience.

Terminology and Pathophysiology

Plantar heel pain is now widely understood as a degenerative load-related disorder rather than a purely inflammatory process. Histopathological and imaging findings support the term plantar fasciopathy in chronic cases, reflecting tissue disorganisation rather than active inflammation.

The plantar fascia functions as a dynamic loadbearing structure, contributing to arch stiffness via the windlass mechanism. Excessive or poorly tolerated load, often in the context of reduced ankle dorsiflexion or altered foot biomechanics, is central to symptom development.

Epidemiology and Burden

- Lifetime prevalence is approximately 10% in the general population
- Most commonly affects adults aged 40–60, but occurs across all age groups
- PHP significantly impacts health-related quality of life, particularly physical function and activity participation
- Recurrence is common, particularly when load is reintroduced faster than tissue capacity is restored

Risk Factors

Consistently reported associations include:

- Increased body mass index and recent weightchange
- Prolonged standing or walking occupations
- Reduced ankle dorsiflexion due to gastrocnemius or Achilles tightness
- Foot posture extremes (pronated or cavus feet), though causality is multifactorial

Heel spurs are common but not causative, appearing frequently in asymptomatic individuals.

Body weight and plantar heel pain

Elevated body mass index (BMI) is a well-established independent risk factor for plantar heel pain, with observational and systematic review data demonstrating a stepwise increase in risk as BMI rises, particularly in non-athletic populations. Biomechanically, higher body weight increases cumulative load through the plantar fascia, contributing to microtrauma, collagen degeneration, increased fascia thickness, and altered tissue stiffness on imaging. Clinical practice guidelines acknowledge the strong association between higher BMI and chronic plantar heel pain; however, evidence that modest, non-surgical weight loss alone produces short-term pain reduction is limited. Exercise-based interventions remain central to management, primarily through targeted stretching and strengthening rather than weight reduction per se. More substantial and sustained weight loss, such as that achieved following bariatric surgery, is associated with significant improvements in plantar fasciitis symptoms, reduced healthcare utilisation, and improved foot-related function. Weight management should therefore be considered a supportive component of a comprehensive, load-informed treatment strategy, rather than a standalone intervention.

Assessment and Diagnosis

Diagnosis is primarily clinical, based on history and examination.

Imaging is not routinely required, but may be appropriate when:

- Symptoms are atypical or refractory
- There is concern for alternative pathology (stress fracture, nerve entrapment)
- Ultrasound can demonstrate increased fascia thickness and structural change

Plain radiographs are useful mainly to exclude bony pathology.

First-Line Management

Strong consensus exists across guidelines and surveys that initial management should focus on education, load modification, and exercise-based care.

Core components:

- Plantar fascia-specific and calf stretching
- Progressive strengthening, particularly of the calf complex
- Footwear advice and prefabricated orthoses, which may reduce pain and improve function 10
- Activity modification, rather than complete rest

A UK survey of healthcare professionals confirms wide adoption of these measures, though sequencing and emphasis vary.

Adjunctive and Escalation Therapies

- **Night splints** may be beneficial in patients with pronounced morning pain
- **Taping** can provide short-term symptom relief
- **Corticosteroid injections** offer short-term pain reduction but carry recognised risks and should be used selectively
- **Extracorporeal shockwave therapy (ESWT)** shows moderate evidence of benefit in chronic cases unresponsive to first-line care

Surgical Considerations

Surgery is required in a small minority (<5–10%) of patients.

Procedures include:

- Partial plantar fasciotomy
- Gastrocnemius recession in cases of demonstrable calf tightness

Outcomes are variable, and surgery should only be considered after 6–12 months of structuredconservative management.

Prognosis

- Approximately 80% improve within 6–9 months

- Around 90% are pain-free by 12 months with appropriate conservative care
- Long-term outcomes are generally favourable, though recurrences are reported

Patient Perspective

Qualitative research highlights the psychological burden of PHP, including frustration, uncertainty, and reduced confidence in movement.

Clear education, realistic timelines, and coherent treatment plans improve adherence and patient satisfaction.

Clinical Implications

- PHP management should prioritise load management, tissue capacity, and patient education
- Over-medicalisation or premature escalation risks prolonging recovery
- Consistency and coherence of care appear more important than the number of modalities used

18. Example products mentioned in this guide

Example products are provided for illustration only and are not endorsements

---

gr8ful® Plantar Fasciitis Night Sock Brace
https://amzn.to/4aSnjqK

Silicone Heel Cup Pads for Plantar Fasciitis
https://amzn.to/4qK7JC7

Arch Support Orthopedic Insoles
https://amzn.to/49wf2qb

Double Strike Insoles - Sorbothane
https://amzn.to/4syMG7h

Plantar Fasciitis Treatment - Plantar Pad
https://amzn.to/49g48WE

Kinetic Muscle Sports tape
https://amzn.to/3NaOKCk

Anti Fatigue Mat
https://amzn.to/3LFI2Uk

Made in United States
North Haven, CT
10 November 2026

22088265R00036